Book Title

Healing Together: Overcoming Domestic Violence as a Family

Authored by Mohamed Tanana

LLM, MHA, MA, MCIArb, NSLS

Table of Contents

FOREWORD

In "Healing Together: Overcoming Domestic Violence as a Family," we embark on a profound journey that addresses one of the most pressing and sensitive issues facing our communities today. Within these pages lies a beacon of hope, a roadmap towards resilience, and a testament to the power of collective healing.

Domestic violence, in its myriad forms, casts a long and dark shadow over countless lives. It knows no boundaries of age, race, gender, or socioeconomic status. Its effects ripple through families, leaving wounds that are both visible and invisible, lasting far beyond the immediate moment of conflict.

Yet, amid the darkness, there exists a glimmer of light – the possibility of transformation, growth, and renewal. This book is a testament to that hope. It is a guide for those navigating the turbulent waters of domestic violence, offering insight, support, and practical strategies for healing.

As we journey through these pages, we will delve into the intricate layers of domestic violence – from its insidious manifestations to its profound impact on individuals, families, and communities.

We will explore the courage it takes to recognize the signs, the resilience it takes to break free from its grip, and the compassion it takes to heal as a family.

Each chapter serves as a stepping stone on the path towards recovery, offering a wealth of knowledge, resources, and guidance along the way. From understanding the complexities of domestic violence to rebuilding trust, fostering communication, and forging a brighter future, this book equips readers with the tools they need to navigate the challenges ahead.

But perhaps most importantly, "Healing Together" reminds us that we are not alone in this journey. Within these pages, we find a community of survivors, advocates, and allies standing shoulder to shoulder, offering support, solidarity, and unwavering hope.

As we embark on this journey together, may we find solace in each other's stories, strength in each other's struggles, and courage in each other's triumphs. For it is only by coming together, as individuals, families, and communities, that we can truly overcome the scourge of domestic violence and pave the way towards a future filled with healing, compassion, and love.

With deep gratitude and unwavering solidarity,

Mohamed Tanana

PREFACE

In the quiet shadows of closed doors, families grapple with a crisis that transcends generations—a struggle against the pervasive specter of domestic violence. "Healing Together" emerges as a beacon of hope amidst this darkness, offering solace, guidance, and a roadmap for collective resilience.

Within the pages of this profound journey, we confront the stark realities of domestic violence, a silent epidemic that knows no bounds of age, gender, or background. Its tendrils reach deep into the fabric of our homes, leaving scars both seen and unseen on the hearts of those it touches.

Yet, amidst the pain, there exists a glimmer of possibility—the prospect of healing, growth, and renewal as a family. "Healing Together" beckons us to embark on this transformative journey, to confront the shadows of our past and forge a future steeped in compassion and understanding.

Through each chapter, we delve into the complexities of domestic violence, from its insidious manifestations to its profound impact on individuals and families. We explore the courage it takes to recognize the signs, the resilience it takes to break free, and the compassion it takes to heal together as a family unit.

But "Healing Together" is more than just a guidebook—it is a testament to the power of community, solidarity, and collective action. It reminds us that we are not alone in our struggles, and that by coming together, we can create a world where every family is free from the shackles of violence.

As we embark on this journey together, may "Healing Together" serve as a source of strength, inspiration, and hope. May it empower us to confront the shadows of domestic violence with courage and compassion, and to forge a future where every home is a sanctuary of safety, respect, and love.

ACKNOWLEDGMENTS

"Healing Together: Overcoming Domestic Violence as a Family" is the culmination of countless efforts, unwavering support, and profound dedication from a multitude of individuals and organizations. As I embark on this journey to confront the shadows of domestic violence, I extend our deepest gratitude to those who have contributed to this endeavor.

First and foremost, I express my heartfelt appreciation to the survivors of domestic violence who bravely shared their stories and experiences. Your resilience, courage, and strength serve as a guiding light, inspiring us to continue the fight for a future free from violence.

To my beloved wife, Alissar, and my children Zahra, Zainab, Mahdi and Zachariah I owe an immeasurable debt of gratitude.

I would like to thank the publisher, for believing in the project and assisting me in spreading awareness regarding domestic violence.

I extend my sincere thanks to the advocates, counselors, and professionals working tirelessly on the front lines of domestic violence prevention and intervention. Your compassion, expertise, and unwavering commitment to supporting survivors are a testament to the power of empathy and solidarity.

To the researchers, scholars, and experts who have dedicated their time and expertise to advancing my understanding of domestic violence, I offer my deepest gratitude. Your insights, knowledge, and contributions have enriched the dialogue surrounding this critical issue and paved the way for meaningful change.

I would also like to thank the organizations and agencies providing vital resources and services to survivors of domestic violence. Your dedication to providing shelter, legal aid, counseling, and support is invaluable in helping individuals and families rebuild their lives.

My gratitude extends to the friends, family members, and allies who have offered their unwavering support and encouragement throughout this journey. Your belief in this mission and your willingness to stand in solidarity with survivors of domestic violence has been a source of strength and inspiration.

Last but certainly not least, I express my deepest appreciation to the readers of "Healing Together." Your willingness to engage with this important dialogue and your commitment to creating a safer, more compassionate world are the driving force behind our collective efforts to overcome domestic violence as a family.

Together, we can confront the shadows of domestic violence with courage, compassion, and solidarity. Thank you for joining us on this transformative journey towards healing and hope.

With deepest gratitude,

Mohamed Tanana

Chapter 1: Understanding Domestic Violence

Defining Domestic Violence

Domestic violence is a pervasive issue that affects families across all walks of life. It is important to understand what constitutes domestic violence in order to address and overcome it. Defining domestic violence is crucial in order to recognize the signs and seek help.

Domestic violence is not limited to physical abuse, although that is often the most visible form. It can also include emotional, psychological, and financial abuse. Emotional abuse may involve manipulation, control, and belittling. Psychological abuse can manifest in threats, intimidation, and isolation. Financial abuse may involve controlling access to money or resources, making it difficult for the victim to leave.

One key aspect of domestic violence is the power and control dynamic. Perpetrators often use their power to exert control over their victims, creating a cycle of abuse that can be difficult to break. This dynamic can manifest in various ways, such as through threats, coercion, or manipulation.

It is important for families to understand that domestic violence is not the fault of the victim. No one deserves to be abused, and it is never acceptable behavior. Seeking help and support is crucial in breaking the cycle of abuse and healing as a family.

By defining domestic violence and understanding its various forms, families can better recognize the signs and take steps towards healing and overcoming this destructive cycle. It is important to educate oneself and seek help from professionals in order to create a safe and healthy environment for all family members. Together, families can work towards breaking the cycle of domestic violence and healing as a unit.

Types of Domestic Violence

Domestic violence can take many different forms, and it is important for families to understand the various types in order to recognize and address them. One common type of domestic violence is physical abuse, which involves using physical force to harm a family member. This can include hitting, punching, kicking, or any other form of physical violence. Physical abuse can leave visible marks on the victim, but it can also cause long-lasting emotional and psychological harm.

Another type of domestic violence is emotional abuse, which involves manipulating, controlling, or belittling a family member in order to exert power and control over them. Emotional abuse can be just as damaging as physical abuse, and it can have a lasting impact on a victim's self-esteem and mental well-being. Examples of emotional abuse include name-calling, constant criticism, and threats of harm.

Financial abuse is another common form of domestic violence that involves controlling a family member's access to money or resources. This can include preventing a partner from working, controlling all of the finances, or withholding money for basic needs. Financial abuse can leave a victim feeling trapped and dependent on their abuser, making it difficult for them to leave the relationship.

Sexual abuse is another type of domestic violence that involves forcing a family member to engage in sexual acts against their will. This can include rape, unwanted sexual touching, or any other form of sexual coercion. Sexual abuse can have a devastating impact on a victim's mental and emotional well-being, and it is important for families to recognize the signs and seek help.

Lastly, psychological abuse is a form of domestic violence that involves using threats, intimidation, or manipulation to control a family member. This can include gaslighting, isolating a victim from friends and family, or using fear to maintain power and control. Psychological abuse can be difficult to detect, but it can have a profound impact on a victim's mental health and well-being. By understanding the different types of domestic violence, families can work together to recognize the signs, seek help, and create a safe and supportive environment for all members.

Impact of Domestic Violence on Families

Domestic violence is a pervasive issue that affects families across all demographics. The impact of domestic violence on families is profound and far-reaching, often causing long-lasting emotional, psychological, and physical harm to all members involved. Children who witness domestic violence are at an increased risk of developing behavioral problems, anxiety, depression, and even engaging in violent behavior themselves. The effects of domestic violence can also manifest in the form of strained relationships, financial instability, and social isolation within the family unit.

One of the most devastating consequences of domestic violence is the breakdown of trust and communication within the family. Victims of domestic violence may feel isolated and ashamed, leading to a reluctance to seek help or support from loved ones. This breakdown in communication can further perpetuate the cycle of violence, as family members may feel unable or unwilling to intervene or offer assistance. In some cases, children may blame themselves for the violence they witness, leading to feelings of guilt, shame, and self-blame.

Domestic violence can also have a significant impact on the physical health of family members. Victims of domestic violence are at a higher risk of developing chronic health conditions, such as heart disease, diabetes, and substance abuse disorders. Children who witness domestic violence may also experience physical health issues, such as headaches, stomachaches, and sleep disturbances. The stress and trauma of living in a violent environment can take a toll on the overall well-being of the entire family, leading to increased healthcare costs and decreased quality of life.

The impact of domestic violence on families can extend beyond the immediate household, affecting relationships with extended family members, friends, and community members. Victims of domestic violence may feel stigmatized or judged by others, leading to feelings of social isolation and alienation. Family members may also experience strained relationships with others as a result of the violence they have experienced or witnessed. This can further compound the trauma and emotional distress experienced by all members of the family, making it difficult to seek help or support from others.

Despite the devastating impact of domestic violence on families, it is possible to heal and overcome the trauma together. By seeking help from trained professionals, such as therapists, counselors, and support groups, families can begin to rebuild trust, communication, and relationships. It is important for families to recognize that they are not alone in their struggles and that there are resources available to help them navigate the challenges of domestic violence. By coming together as a family and supporting one another through the healing process, families can begin to break the cycle of violence and create a safe and nurturing environment for all members to thrive. Healing together is possible, and with the right support and resources, families can overcome domestic violence and create a brighter future for themselves and their loved ones.

Chapter 2: Recognizing the Signs of Domestic Violence

Physical Signs

In the midst of domestic violence, there are often physical signs that can indicate abuse is occurring within a family. These signs may not always be immediately visible, but it is important for families to be aware of them in order to seek help and support. Physical signs of domestic violence can include bruises, cuts, burns, or broken bones. These injuries may be explained away as accidents, but if they occur frequently or seem suspicious, it is important to consider the possibility of domestic violence.

It is crucial for families to pay attention to any unexplained physical injuries that occur within the household. These injuries may not only be limited to the victim of the abuse, but also to children or other family members who may be caught in the crossfire. If you notice frequent injuries or injuries that seem suspicious, it is important to seek help and support from a trusted source, such as a domestic violence hotline or local shelter.

In addition to physical injuries, there may also be other physical signs of domestic violence that are less obvious. These signs can include changes in behavior or appearance, such as weight loss, fatigue, or changes in sleep patterns. Victims of domestic violence may also experience physical symptoms such as headaches, stomachaches, or other unexplained pains. These physical signs can be indicators of the stress and trauma that often accompany domestic violence.

It is important for families to be aware of these physical signs of domestic violence in order to provide support and assistance to those who may be experiencing abuse. By recognizing the physical signs of abuse, families can take steps to address the situation and seek help for themselves or their loved ones. It is essential for families to come together and support each other in overcoming domestic violence and creating a safe and healthy environment for all members.

By understanding and recognizing the physical signs of domestic violence, families can take the first step towards healing and overcoming the cycle of abuse. It is important for families to work together to create a safe and supportive environment where all members can thrive and heal from the trauma of domestic violence. By acknowledging the physical signs of abuse and seeking help and support, families can begin the journey towards healing together.

Emotional Signs

In the journey of healing from domestic violence as a family, it is crucial to recognize and understand the emotional signs that may manifest in both the survivors and the perpetrators. These emotional signs can serve as important indicators of the impact of the abuse and the need for intervention and support. By being aware of these signs, families can better navigate the healing process and work towards a healthier and safer future.

One of the key emotional signs to look out for in survivors of domestic violence is fear. Survivors may exhibit signs of anxiety, hypervigilance, and a sense of constant fear for their safety and the safety of their loved ones. This fear can be paralyzing and can prevent survivors from seeking help or speaking out about the abuse. It is important for families to create a safe and supportive environment where survivors feel empowered to share their experiences and seek the help they need.

Guilt and shame are also common emotional signs that survivors of domestic violence may experience. Survivors may blame themselves for the abuse or feel ashamed of what they have endured. This can lead to feelings of worthlessness and self-doubt, making it difficult for survivors to rebuild their sense of self-worth and confidence.

Families can help survivors by offering reassurance, validation, and unconditional support, and by helping them recognize that the abuse is not their fault.

On the other hand, perpetrators of domestic violence may exhibit emotional signs such as anger, control, and manipulation. Perpetrators may use these emotions to maintain power and control over their victims, and to justify their abusive behavior. It is important for families to recognize these signs and to hold perpetrators accountable for their actions. By addressing these emotional signs and behaviors, families can create a safer and healthier environment for everyone involved.

In healing from domestic violence as a family, it is important to remember that emotional signs are not always visible on the surface. Each individual may experience and express their emotions differently, and it is important to be patient and understanding as everyone navigates their own healing journey. By creating a supportive and non-judgmental environment, families can help each other process and heal from the emotional impact of domestic violence, and work towards a future free from abuse.

Behavioral Signs

In order to effectively address domestic violence within a family unit, it is essential to be able to recognize and understand the behavioral signs that may indicate the presence of abuse. These signs can manifest in a variety of ways and it is crucial for families to be aware of these indicators in order to intervene and seek help as needed.

One common behavioral sign of domestic violence is a noticeable change in the demeanor or behavior of the victim. This may include increased anxiety, fearfulness, or withdrawal from social activities. It is important for family members to be attuned to these changes and to offer support and assistance to the individual experiencing abuse.

Another behavioral sign to look out for is a pattern of controlling or manipulative behavior from one partner towards the other. This can manifest in various ways, such as monitoring the victim's movements, restricting their access to finances, or isolating them from friends and family. Recognizing these behaviors as early warning signs of abuse can help families intervene before the situation escalates.

In some cases, children may also exhibit behavioral signs of domestic violence within the family. This can include changes in mood or behavior, difficulty concentrating at school, or physical symptoms such as stomachaches or headaches. It is important for parents and caregivers to be attentive to these signs and to create a safe and supportive environment for children to express their feelings and concerns.

By being aware of the behavioral signs of domestic violence and taking proactive steps to address them, families can work together to overcome abuse and create a healthier and safer environment for all members. It is essential for families to communicate openly and honestly about these issues, seek help from professionals when needed, and support each other in the journey towards healing and recovery.

Chapter 3: Breaking the Cycle of Domestic Violence

Seeking Help

Seeking help is a crucial step in overcoming domestic violence as a family. It can be a daunting and overwhelming process, but it is important to remember that you are not alone. There are numerous resources available to support you and your loved ones through this difficult time. Whether you are experiencing abuse or know someone who is, reaching out for help is the first step towards healing and creating a safe environment for your family.

One of the most important things to remember when seeking help is that there is no shame in asking for assistance. Domestic violence is a complex issue that can have lasting effects on individuals and families. By reaching out for help, you are taking a brave and necessary step towards breaking the cycle of abuse and creating a healthier environment for yourself and your loved ones. Remember, you deserve to be safe and supported, and there are people who are ready and willing to help you through this difficult time.

When seeking help for domestic violence, it is important to reach out to trusted professionals who are trained to support individuals and families experiencing abuse. This may include domestic violence shelters, counseling services, legal resources, and support groups. These organizations can provide you with the tools and resources you need to navigate the complexities of domestic violence and create a safety plan for yourself and your family. By seeking help from trained professionals, you can ensure that you are receiving the support and guidance you need to move forward in a healthy and safe way.

In addition to professional resources, it is also important to reach out to friends and family members who can offer emotional support and guidance. Trusted loved ones can provide you with a listening ear, a shoulder to lean on, and practical assistance in times of crisis. By building a strong support network of friends and family members, you can create a sense of community and connection that can help you through the healing process. Remember, you do not have to face domestic violence alone – there are people who care about you and want to help you through this difficult time.

Remember, seeking help is not a sign of weakness – it is a sign of strength and courage. By reaching out for support, you are taking an important step towards creating a safe and healthy environment for yourself and your loved ones. Whether you are experiencing abuse or know someone who is, there are resources available to help you through this difficult time. By seeking help from trusted professionals, building a strong support network, and creating a safety plan, you can begin the healing process and create a brighter future for yourself and your family.

Creating a Safety Plan

One of the most important steps in overcoming domestic violence as a family is to create a safety plan. A safety plan is a personalized, practical plan that outlines steps to take in order to stay safe in dangerous situations. It is crucial for families experiencing domestic violence to have a safety plan in place in order to protect themselves and their loved ones from harm.

When creating a safety plan, it is important to consider the specific needs and circumstances of your family. This may include identifying safe places to go in an emergency, developing a code word or signal to communicate distress, and establishing a support network of trusted friends, family members, or community resources. It is also important to include children in the safety planning process and ensure that they understand what to do in case of an emergency.

In addition to physical safety, it is also important to consider emotional and psychological safety when creating a safety plan. This may involve seeking counseling or therapy for yourself and your children, setting boundaries with the abuser, and practicing self-care techniques to manage stress and anxiety. Remember that your emotional well-being is just as important as your physical safety, and it is okay to prioritize your own needs and feelings.

It is important to regularly review and update your safety plan as needed. As circumstances change and new challenges arise, it is crucial to reassess your safety plan and make any necessary adjustments. This may involve seeking additional support from a domestic violence advocate, therapist, or other professional who can help you navigate the complexities of domestic violence and provide guidance on how to stay safe.

Remember, creating a safety plan is an empowering step towards healing and overcoming domestic violence as a family. By taking proactive measures to protect yourself and your loved ones, you are demonstrating resilience and strength in the face of adversity. You are not alone in this journey, and there are resources and support available to help you navigate the challenges of domestic violence and build a safer, healthier future for yourself and your family.

Legal Options

When dealing with domestic violence, it is important for families to understand the legal options available to them. Seeking legal help can provide protection and support for victims of domestic violence, as well as hold the abuser accountable for their actions. There are several legal avenues that families can explore to ensure their safety and well-being.

One option for families experiencing domestic violence is to obtain a restraining order or protection order. This legal document can prohibit the abuser from contacting or coming near the victim and their family members. It serves as a legal tool to prevent further abuse and harassment. It is important for families to understand the process of obtaining a restraining order and the steps involved in filing for one.

Another legal option for families is to seek help from law enforcement. Victims of domestic violence can report abuse to the police, who can then investigate the situation and take appropriate action. Law enforcement can provide immediate protection and support for victims, as well as assist in holding the abuser accountable for their actions. It is important for families to know that they can reach out to the police for help in times of crisis.

In addition to restraining orders and law enforcement intervention, families can also seek legal assistance from domestic violence advocacy organizations or attorneys. These professionals can provide guidance and support in navigating the legal system and obtaining the necessary protection for victims of domestic violence. They can also help families understand their rights and options when it comes to seeking legal recourse against the abuser.

Overall, understanding the legal options available to families experiencing domestic violence is crucial in ensuring their safety and well-being. By seeking help from law enforcement, obtaining restraining orders, and seeking legal assistance, families can take proactive steps to protect themselves and hold abusers accountable for their actions. It is important for families to know that they are not alone and that there are resources available to help them navigate the legal system and overcome domestic violence.

Chapter 4: Healing as a Family

Family Therapy

Family therapy is an essential component in overcoming domestic violence as a family unit. It provides a safe space for family members to address and work through the underlying issues that contribute to the cycle of violence. By engaging in therapy together, families can learn effective communication skills, healthy coping mechanisms, and strategies to build stronger, more supportive relationships.

One of the key benefits of family therapy is that it allows all members of the family to have a voice and be heard. This is especially important in cases of domestic violence, where power and control dynamics can silence victims and perpetuate harmful behaviors. In therapy, each family member is given the opportunity to share their perspective, feelings, and experiences in a nonjudgmental and supportive environment.

Family therapy also helps families develop a deeper understanding of the dynamics of domestic violence and how it impacts each member individually and as a whole. Through guided conversations and exercises, families can explore the root causes of violence, identify triggers, and develop strategies to break the cycle of abuse. By gaining insight into the underlying issues, families can work towards healing and creating a safer, more peaceful environment for everyone involved.

Another important aspect of family therapy is building trust and fostering healthy relationships within the family unit. Many families impacted by domestic violence struggle with trust issues, fear, and feelings of isolation. Through therapy, families can learn how to rebuild trust, set boundaries, and establish open lines of communication. This can help family members feel more connected, supported, and valued, ultimately strengthening their bond and resilience.

In conclusion, family therapy is a powerful tool in overcoming domestic violence and rebuilding healthy, thriving family relationships. By addressing the root causes of violence, fostering open communication, and building trust, families can heal together and create a safe and supportive environment for all members. If you are experiencing domestic violence in your family, consider seeking out a qualified family therapist who can help you navigate this challenging journey towards healing and transformation.

Individual Therapy

Individual therapy is an essential component of the healing process for those who have experienced domestic violence. In this subchapter, we will explore the benefits of individual therapy for both survivors and perpetrators of domestic violence. Through individual therapy, individuals can process their trauma in a safe and supportive environment, allowing them to heal and move forward in their lives.

For survivors of domestic violence, individual therapy provides a space to address the emotional and psychological effects of their experiences. Therapy can help survivors work through feelings of guilt, shame, and fear, and develop healthy coping mechanisms to manage their emotions. By exploring their past experiences with a trained therapist, survivors can gain insight into how their past trauma has impacted their present behavior and relationships.

Individual therapy can also be beneficial for perpetrators of domestic violence. By examining the root causes of their abusive behavior, perpetrators can begin to understand and change their harmful patterns. Through therapy, perpetrators can learn healthy communication skills, anger management techniques, and strategies for resolving conflicts in a non-violent manner. Therapy can also help perpetrators address any underlying mental health issues that may be contributing to their abusive behavior.

In individual therapy, survivors and perpetrators can work towards healing and growth on their own terms. Therapy provides a safe and confidential space for individuals to explore their thoughts and feelings without fear of judgment or retribution. Through therapy, individuals can build self-awareness, self-esteem, and resilience, empowering them to break free from the cycle of violence and create a healthier future for themselves and their families.

Overall, individual therapy is a valuable tool for those who have experienced domestic violence. By seeking help from a qualified therapist, survivors and perpetrators can begin the healing process and work towards a future free from violence. Through individual therapy, individuals can gain insight, develop coping skills, and build healthier relationships, ultimately creating a more peaceful and loving environment for themselves and their families.

Support Groups

Support groups can be a valuable resource for families experiencing domestic violence. These groups provide a safe space for individuals to share their experiences, seek advice, and receive emotional support from others who have gone through similar situations. By connecting with others who understand their struggles, families can feel less isolated and more empowered to make positive changes in their lives.

Attending a support group can also help families learn more about domestic violence, its effects, and the resources available to them. Many support groups offer educational materials, workshops, and guest speakers who can provide valuable information on topics such as safety planning, legal rights, and healthy relationships. By gaining knowledge and insight from these sources, families can better understand their options and make informed decisions about their future.

In addition to providing emotional support and education, support groups can also help families build a sense of community and connection. By forming relationships with other group members, families can create a network of support that extends beyond the group meetings. These connections can provide a sense of belonging, reduce feelings of shame or stigma, and offer opportunities for socializing and recreation.

Support groups can also serve as a valuable resource for families seeking professional help. Many support groups have partnerships with local organizations, shelters, and counseling services that can provide additional support and guidance. By connecting with these resources, families can access the help they need to address their specific needs and concerns.

Overall, support groups can be a powerful tool for families healing from domestic violence. By providing a safe space for sharing, learning, and connecting, these groups can help families navigate their experiences, build resilience, and move forward on their journey to healing and recovery.

Chapter 5: Rebuilding Trust and Communication

Rebuilding Trust

Rebuilding trust after experiencing domestic violence can be a long and challenging process for families. It is important to remember that trust is fragile and can take time to rebuild. However, with patience, understanding, and dedication, it is possible to heal together as a family.

One of the first steps in rebuilding trust is open and honest communication. Family members should feel comfortable expressing their feelings and concerns in a safe and non-judgmental environment. This can help to rebuild trust by creating a sense of transparency and understanding within the family unit.

Another important aspect of rebuilding trust is setting boundaries and expectations. It is crucial for family members to establish clear boundaries and expectations for behavior moving forward. This can help to create a sense of safety and predictability within the family, which is essential for rebuilding trust.

It is also important for families to seek outside support and resources during the process of rebuilding trust. Therapy, support groups, and other resources can provide families with the tools and guidance they need to navigate the challenges of healing together after experiencing domestic violence.

Ultimately, rebuilding trust as a family is a journey that requires time, patience, and dedication. By prioritizing open communication, setting boundaries, seeking outside support, and approaching the process with empathy and understanding, families can work towards healing together and rebuilding trust in a healthy and positive way.

Improving Communication

Improving communication is essential for families who are trying to overcome domestic violence. When there is open and honest communication within the family, it can help to break down barriers and create a safe space for everyone to express their thoughts and feelings. By improving communication, families can work together to address the root causes of domestic violence and find healthier ways to resolve conflicts.

One way to improve communication within a family affected by domestic violence is to practice active listening. This means truly listening to what the other person is saying without interrupting or judging them. By actively listening, family members can feel heard and understood, which can help build trust and strengthen relationships.

Another important aspect of improving communication is being able to express emotions in a healthy way. Many times, domestic violence stems from a lack of effective communication about emotions and feelings. By teaching family members how to express themselves in a constructive manner, it can help reduce the likelihood of conflicts escalating into violence.

Setting boundaries and expectations for communication is also key in improving communication within a family affected by domestic violence. By establishing ground rules for how family members should communicate with each other, it can help create a sense of safety and respect within the family unit. This can also help prevent misunderstandings and conflicts from escalating.

Ultimately, improving communication within a family affected by domestic violence requires effort and commitment from all family members. By practicing active listening, expressing emotions in a healthy way, and setting boundaries for communication, families can work together to create a safe and supportive environment where everyone feels valued and respected. This can help break the cycle of violence and create a foundation for healing and growth as a family.

Setting Boundaries

Setting boundaries is a crucial aspect of healing from domestic violence as a family. It is important to establish clear and healthy boundaries in order to create a safe and supportive environment for everyone involved. By setting boundaries, you are defining what is acceptable behavior and what is not, which can help prevent further abuse and promote respectful communication within the family.

One way to set boundaries is by clearly communicating your needs and expectations to each other. This can involve discussing what behaviors are unacceptable, such as yelling, name-calling, or physical violence. By expressing your boundaries in a calm and assertive manner, you are establishing healthy communication patterns that can help prevent conflicts from escalating.

It is also important to set boundaries with external factors that may contribute to the cycle of abuse. This can include limiting contact with individuals who may enable or support the abusive behavior, such as friends or family members who dismiss or minimize the abuse. By creating a supportive network of individuals who respect your boundaries and offer positive reinforcement, you can strengthen your family's resilience and ability to heal together.

In addition to communicating boundaries, it is important to enforce them consistently. This may involve setting consequences for violating boundaries, such as temporarily removing yourself from a situation that is becoming unsafe or seeking professional help if necessary. By holding each other accountable for respecting boundaries, you are creating a culture of mutual respect and trust within the family.

Ultimately, setting boundaries is an ongoing process that requires patience, communication, and self-reflection. It is important to regularly check in with each other to ensure that boundaries are being respected and adjust them as needed. By prioritizing the well-being and safety of each family member, you are taking a proactive step towards healing together from the impact of domestic violence.

Chapter 6: Moving Forward

Setting Goals for the Future

Setting goals for the future is an important step in the healing process for families who have experienced domestic violence. By creating a vision for what they want their lives to look like moving forward, families can begin to take positive steps towards a brighter future. Setting goals allows families to focus on what is most important to them and helps them to stay motivated and hopeful during difficult times.

When setting goals for the future, it is important for families to be realistic and specific. Setting vague or unrealistic goals can lead to feelings of frustration and disappointment. Instead, families should take the time to think carefully about what they want to achieve and create clear, achievable milestones along the way. By breaking larger goals down into smaller, more manageable steps, families can make progress towards their vision for the future.

In addition to being realistic and specific, goals should also be measurable. This means that families should be able to track their progress towards their goals and celebrate their achievements along the way. By setting measurable goals, families can stay motivated and see the tangible results of their hard work and dedication. Whether it is improving communication, finding a new home, or seeking counseling, families can track their progress and adjust their goals as needed.

It is also important for families to set goals that are meaningful and aligned with their values. By setting goals that are truly important to them, families can stay committed and motivated, even when faced with challenges. Whether it is creating a safe and loving home environment, building stronger relationships, or pursuing education and career opportunities, families should choose goals that reflect their deepest desires and aspirations for the future.

Ultimately, setting goals for the future is an empowering and transformative process for families who have experienced domestic violence. By creating a clear vision for what they want their lives to look like, families can begin to take control of their own destinies and build a brighter future together. Through setting realistic, specific, measurable, and meaningful goals, families can stay focused, motivated, and hopeful as they work towards healing and overcoming the impact of domestic violence.

Building a Support System

One of the most crucial aspects of overcoming domestic violence as a family is building a strong support system. This network of individuals can provide emotional, practical, and financial assistance during difficult times. It is essential for families experiencing domestic violence to reach out and connect with people who can offer support and guidance.

Family members should start by reaching out to trusted friends, family members, or religious leaders who can provide a listening ear and offer comfort and advice. It is important to confide in individuals who are non-judgmental and who will support the family in making positive changes. Building a support system also involves seeking out professional help, such as counselors, therapists, or support groups, who can provide guidance and resources for healing.

In addition to seeking support from friends and professionals, families experiencing domestic violence can also benefit from connecting with community resources. This may include local shelters, hotlines, or advocacy groups that specialize in supporting victims of domestic violence. By reaching out to these organizations, families can access additional resources, such as legal assistance, housing options, and safety planning.

It is important for families to remember that they are not alone in their journey to overcome domestic violence. By building a support system, they can create a strong network of individuals who are dedicated to helping them heal and move forward. By reaching out for help and connecting with others who have experienced similar challenges, families can find hope and strength in knowing that they are not alone.

Overall, building a support system is essential for families to heal and overcome domestic violence. By connecting with friends, family members, professionals, and community resources, families can access the support and resources they need to navigate the challenges of domestic violence. With a strong support system in place, families can begin the healing process and work towards creating a safe and stable environment for themselves and their loved ones.

Practicing Self-Care

Practicing self-care is crucial for families who have experienced domestic violence. It is important for both the survivors and their children to prioritize their mental, emotional, and physical well-being in order to heal and move forward from the trauma they have experienced. Self-care can take many forms, from engaging in activities that bring joy and relaxation to seeking professional help and support.

One of the first steps in practicing self-care is recognizing the impact that domestic violence has had on you and your family. It is important to acknowledge the pain and trauma that you have experienced and to give yourself permission to feel and process these emotions. This can be a difficult and painful process, but it is essential for healing and moving forward.

Self-care also involves setting boundaries and prioritizing your own needs. This may mean saying no to activities or people that drain your energy or trigger negative emotions. It may also mean seeking out therapy or counseling to work through the trauma and develop healthy coping mechanisms. Taking care of yourself is not selfish - it is necessary in order to be able to care for your family and support them through their healing journey.

Engaging in self-care activities can help families build resilience and cope with the challenges of healing from domestic violence. This may include practicing mindfulness and meditation, engaging in physical exercise, spending time in nature, or pursuing creative outlets such as art or music. Finding activities that bring joy and relaxation can help families reduce stress and build a sense of connection and support.

Ultimately, practicing self-care is a vital component of healing from domestic violence as a family. By prioritizing your own well-being and taking steps to care for yourself, you can build resilience, cope with the trauma, and support your family in their healing journey. Remember, you deserve to prioritize your own needs and take care of yourself in order to heal and move forward as a family.

Chapter 7: Resources for Families Affected by Domestic Violence

Hotlines and Helplines

Hotlines and helplines are essential resources for families experiencing domestic violence. These services provide immediate support and assistance to individuals in crisis, offering a lifeline for those who may feel trapped or alone in their situation. By reaching out to a hotline or helpline, families can access valuable information, resources, and support to help them navigate the challenges of domestic violence.

One of the key benefits of hotlines and helplines is their 24/7 availability. Whether it's the middle of the night or a holiday weekend, families can always reach out for help when they need it most. This around-the-clock support ensures that no one has to face domestic violence alone, and that help is always just a phone call away.

Hotlines and helplines also provide a safe and confidential space for families to discuss their experiences and seek guidance. Trained professionals and advocates are available to listen, offer support, and connect families with additional resources such as shelters, counseling services, and legal assistance. By calling a hotline or helpline, families can take the first step towards healing and creating a safer environment for themselves and their loved ones.

In addition to providing immediate support, hotlines and helplines can also help families develop safety plans and explore their options for leaving an abusive situation. These services can offer advice on how to stay safe, connect families with local resources, and provide guidance on how to navigate the complex legal and social services systems. By utilizing the expertise of hotline and helpline staff, families can make informed decisions about their next steps and begin to rebuild their lives free from violence.

Overall, hotlines and helplines play a crucial role in supporting families affected by domestic violence. By reaching out for help, families can access the resources and support they need to heal, stay safe, and break free from the cycle of abuse. It's important for families to know that they are not alone and that help is available whenever they need it. By utilizing hotlines and helplines, families can take an important step towards healing together as they overcome domestic violence.

Shelters and Safe Houses

Shelters and safe houses play a crucial role in providing protection and support for families experiencing domestic violence. These facilities offer a safe haven for individuals and families to escape from abusive situations and begin the healing process. In times of crisis, shelters can offer temporary housing, counseling services, legal assistance, and resources to help survivors rebuild their lives. It is important for families to know that they are not alone and that there are organizations and shelters dedicated to helping them through this difficult time.

When seeking refuge in a shelter or safe house, families can expect to find a supportive and understanding environment where their safety is the top priority. Trained staff members are available around the clock to provide guidance, support, and resources to help families navigate the challenges of leaving an abusive relationship. Shelters also offer a sense of community and connection, allowing survivors to share their stories and experiences with others who have gone through similar situations. This sense of solidarity can be empowering and validating for families who may feel isolated or alone in their struggles.

In addition to providing immediate safety and shelter, these facilities also offer a range of services to help families rebuild their lives and move forward from the trauma of domestic violence. Counseling and therapy services are available to help survivors process their experiences, heal from emotional wounds, and develop coping strategies for the future. Legal advocacy and support can help families navigate the complexities of the legal system, obtain protection orders, and access resources to secure their safety and well-being. Shelters and safe houses are equipped to assist families with practical needs such as housing, employment, childcare, and financial assistance as they transition to a life free from abuse.

It is important for families to know that seeking help from a shelter or safe house is not a sign of weakness, but rather a courageous step towards reclaiming their lives and breaking the cycle of violence. By reaching out for support, families are taking a stand against abuse and prioritizing their safety and well-being. Shelters and safe houses are a lifeline for families in crisis, providing a safe and nurturing environment where healing can begin. No family should have to endure domestic violence alone, and shelters are here to offer the support and resources needed to overcome this difficult chapter and move towards a brighter future.

In conclusion, shelters and safe houses are essential resources for families experiencing domestic violence, offering safety, support, and empowerment in times of crisis. By seeking help from these facilities, families can access a range of services to help them heal, rebuild, and move forward from abuse. It is important for families to know that they are not alone and that help is available to support them through this challenging time. Shelters and safe houses play a vital role in breaking the cycle of violence and empowering families to create a future free from abuse. Healing together as a family is possible with the support of shelters and safe houses.

Legal Aid and Advocacy Organizations

Legal Aid and Advocacy Organizations play a crucial role in supporting families affected by domestic violence. These organizations provide free or low-cost legal services to individuals who are unable to afford representation. They help survivors navigate the legal system, obtain protective orders, and secure custody of their children. By partnering with these organizations, families can access the resources and support they need to break free from abusive situations and rebuild their lives.

One of the primary benefits of working with Legal Aid and Advocacy Organizations is the expertise they bring to the table. These organizations employ skilled attorneys and advocates who specialize in domestic violence cases. They understand the complexities of the legal system and can provide invaluable guidance to survivors as they seek justice and protection. By leveraging their knowledge and experience, families can increase their chances of securing favorable outcomes in court proceedings and other legal matters.

In addition to legal representation, Legal Aid and Advocacy Organizations offer a range of support services to families impacted by domestic violence. This may include counseling, support groups, and referrals to other community resources. By addressing the emotional and practical needs of survivors, these organizations help families heal and move forward in a positive direction. They create a safe and empowering environment where individuals can share their experiences, receive validation, and access the help they need to thrive.

Furthermore, Legal Aid and Advocacy Organizations play a key role in advocating for policy changes and systemic reforms to better protect survivors of domestic violence. Through their lobbying efforts and partnerships with lawmakers, these organizations work to strengthen laws and policies that address domestic violence and hold abusers accountable. By amplifying the voices of survivors and raising awareness about the issue, they contribute to a more just and equitable society where all families can live free from violence and fear.

In conclusion, Legal Aid and Advocacy Organizations are invaluable allies for families impacted by domestic violence. By providing legal representation, support services, and advocacy efforts, these organizations empower survivors to seek justice, heal from trauma, and rebuild their lives. Families can benefit greatly from partnering with these organizations and accessing the resources and support they offer. Together, we can work towards a future where domestic violence is eradicated, and all families can thrive in safety and peace.

Chapter 8: Conclusion

Celebrating Progress

In the subchapter titled "Celebrating Progress" from the book "Healing Together: Overcoming Domestic Violence as a Family," we want to acknowledge and celebrate the steps that families affected by domestic violence have taken towards healing and recovery. It is important to recognize that progress, no matter how small, is a significant achievement in the journey towards breaking free from the cycle of abuse.

One way that families can celebrate progress is by reflecting on how far they have come since the beginning of their healing journey. Whether it is seeking help from a therapist, joining a support group, or implementing safety plans, each step taken towards healing is a reason to celebrate. By acknowledging the progress made, families can boost their confidence and motivation to continue working towards a violence-free future.

Another way to celebrate progress is by setting achievable goals and milestones for the family to work towards together. These goals can be as simple as communicating openly and honestly with each other, practicing self-care, or establishing healthy boundaries. By setting goals and celebrating when they are achieved, families can build a sense of accomplishment and unity as they navigate the challenges of overcoming domestic violence.

Celebrating progress can also involve recognizing and appreciating the efforts of each family member in the healing process. It is important to acknowledge the courage and resilience it takes to confront and address the trauma of domestic violence. By expressing gratitude and support for each other, families can strengthen their bonds and create a positive and nurturing environment for healing.

Ultimately, celebrating progress is about recognizing the strength and determination of families as they work towards a violence-free future. By acknowledging and celebrating the steps taken towards healing, families can build resilience, restore trust, and create a safe and supportive environment for each other. As families continue on their journey towards healing together, it is important to celebrate each milestone, no matter how small, as a testament to their strength and commitment to breaking free from the cycle of abuse.

Looking Towards a Brighter Future

In this subchapter, we want to emphasize the importance of looking towards a brighter future for families who have experienced domestic violence. While the past may have been filled with pain and trauma, it is essential to focus on healing and moving forward as a family unit. By working together and supporting each other, families can overcome the challenges of domestic violence and create a brighter future for themselves and their loved ones.

One of the first steps towards a brighter future is seeking help and support. Domestic violence can have lasting effects on individuals and families, and it is crucial to reach out for assistance from professionals who can provide guidance and resources. By seeking therapy, counseling, or support groups, families can begin the healing process and work towards creating a safer and healthier environment for everyone involved.

Another important aspect of looking towards a brighter future is fostering open communication within the family. By creating a safe space for everyone to share their thoughts and feelings, families can address any issues that may arise and work together to find solutions. This can help build trust and strengthen relationships, ultimately leading to a more positive and supportive family dynamic.

Setting goals and creating a plan for the future can also help families move forward from the trauma of domestic violence. By identifying specific objectives and taking small steps towards achieving them, families can regain a sense of control and empowerment. Whether it's pursuing education, finding stable housing, or rebuilding relationships, having a clear vision for the future can provide hope and motivation for families to continue on their healing journey.

In conclusion, looking towards a brighter future after experiencing domestic violence is possible with the right support and mindset. By seeking help, fostering open communication, setting goals, and working together as a family, individuals can overcome the challenges of the past and create a positive and thriving future for themselves and their loved ones. It is never too late to start the healing process and work towards a brighter future for the entire family.

Continuing the Journey of Healing Together

Continuing the journey of healing together is a crucial step for families who have experienced domestic violence. It is important to recognize that healing is not a linear process, and it often takes time and effort to work through the trauma and rebuild trust within the family unit. By committing to this journey together, families can find strength in each other and support one another in their healing process.

One key aspect of continuing the journey of healing together is open and honest communication. It is essential for family members to be able to express their feelings and emotions in a safe and non-judgmental environment. By creating a space for open dialogue, families can begin to understand each other's experiences and work towards healing as a collective unit.

Another important aspect of healing together is seeking professional help and support. There are many resources available for families who have experienced domestic violence, including therapy, support groups, and counseling services. By seeking help from trained professionals, families can gain valuable insights and tools to navigate the healing process and move forward in a positive direction.

In addition to professional help, it is also important for families to support each other in their healing journey. This may involve setting boundaries, practicing self-care, and showing empathy and understanding towards one another. By offering support and encouragement, families can create a sense of unity and strength that will help them overcome the challenges of healing from domestic violence.

Overall, continuing the journey of healing together is a process that requires patience, understanding, and commitment from all family members. By working together, families can create a safe and nurturing environment where healing can take place, and where they can rebuild trust, resilience, and love. Healing from domestic violence is possible, and by coming together as a family, families can overcome the trauma and create a brighter future for themselves and their loved ones.

www.ingramcontent.com/pod-product-compliance
Lightning Source LLC
Chambersburg PA
CBHW051704250726
48653CB00007B/2840